Table of Contents

"Success usually comes to those who are too busy to be looking for it."

Henry David Thoreau

Introduction

I'm the creator and author of "*Going from Fat to Thin In 30 Days*". I'm your trainer Darrick Bynum. I'm not here to give you my resume. I don't want to bore you or give you a bunch of info that you won't remember or that you frankly don't care about. How many times have you picked up a weight loss book and wondered "what does that mean" or "who cares?" "Just teach me how to get rid of these rolls?" I'm going to talk to you as if you are a

5-year old. I hope that does not insult you but rather helps you understand that in the next 30 days your body will change. I will coach you all the way through your weight loss journey. Let's get our gluteus maximus off the couch and rip your bodies to a flatter belly. Why do we need to rip our bodies? Well, do you want to keep struggling to hide that muffin top? Don't you want to enjoy a long healthy life with a slimmer sexier you? So dump the soda pop, potato chips, cookies, and all the sugar and sweets. Remember that sugar is our enemy. It only causes your favorite clothes not to fit anymore. If I see you eating junk food, I'm going to call you a muffin top. If you want to eat junk food then go right ahead and eat the junk food, but you won't become a sexier new you that way. I'm just teasing, but let's get serious. It's very important that you get a journal. Make sure to keep record of everything that you eat. Even the junk food needs to be recorded. When you look back at your entries you can push yourself to try harder in changing those unhealthy fat-cell-growing-habits. I always see my clients hide their food when they see me coming. The point here is that we crave junk food and we love to eat it.

However, we don't acknowledge that the way we eat is a problem. I call this the meet and greet approach. You meet the fat by acknowledging there is a problem. You greet the fat by being a great hostess to the fat, by melting it away. So let's bust and melt the fat away by getting down to business.

"If you are not willing to risk the usual, you will have to settle for the ordinary."

Jim Rohn

"It is not the strongest of the species that survive, nor the most intelligent, but the one most responsive to change."

Charles Darwin

You really need to STOP making excuses!!

Do you always procrastinate by saying "Oh, I will just work out tomorrow"? Then tomorrow comes and you put it off promising that you will start your workout next week. Making empty promises to a healthier body is only prolonging melting off that muffin top. Stop being a procrastinator and you will get the results you want for your body!

Call to action

Put your words into action. Do what you say you are going to do and stop making those lame excuses. You have to plan for a day that you can commit to working out, write that down, and place reminders everywhere possible. Start by writing it down in a calendar and posting little notes in your bathroom. I recommend posting your first day workout on Facebook. The reason for this is that when you post it on Facebook, your family and friends will also support you!

We all know it feels good to get attention because it makes you feel loved, and that's why I'm going to train you. I know life throws curveballs, but you have to be strong. This new lifestyle will change your life. It doesn't matter who you are, I care, and that's why I'm offering this book to you at a very nominal price. I'm right by your side every step of the way and when you feel like eating a pizza and quitting then try to remember the following: "You're a muffin top!" Just kidding! When the going gets tough you will get tougher, something like that, no I'm playing with you. What doesn't kill you only makes you stronger, I live by that, and you should as well. We all have problems but keep in mind there are people in worse situations then you are. So remember you are not alone at all. Whenever I get down about something, I like to pray to God and ask him to give me the strength I need. I can tell you we live in a cruel world, but you can change and I have faith in you. That's right, I said that loud and clear, I have faith in you. Don't ever think you can't do something, because you can. So drop and give me 100 pushups. Yes, you heard me right, and don't get up until I tell you to recover.

You probably think I'm crazy. Hey, maybe I am, but you really do need to distance yourself far away from negativity. It's a shame to only hear about people who are struggling. How often are you around negative people? Negativity is an enemy to life and will give you nothing but negative results. It drains your body and slows down the fat melting process. We have to change the way we live and keep ourselves away from the negativity. Find the things that you love, keep those things in mean, and no, I'm not talking about your favorite burger. Now that we took the garbage out, we are free and clear of all the negative vibes in life, and I can push you to a better, healthier lifestyle.

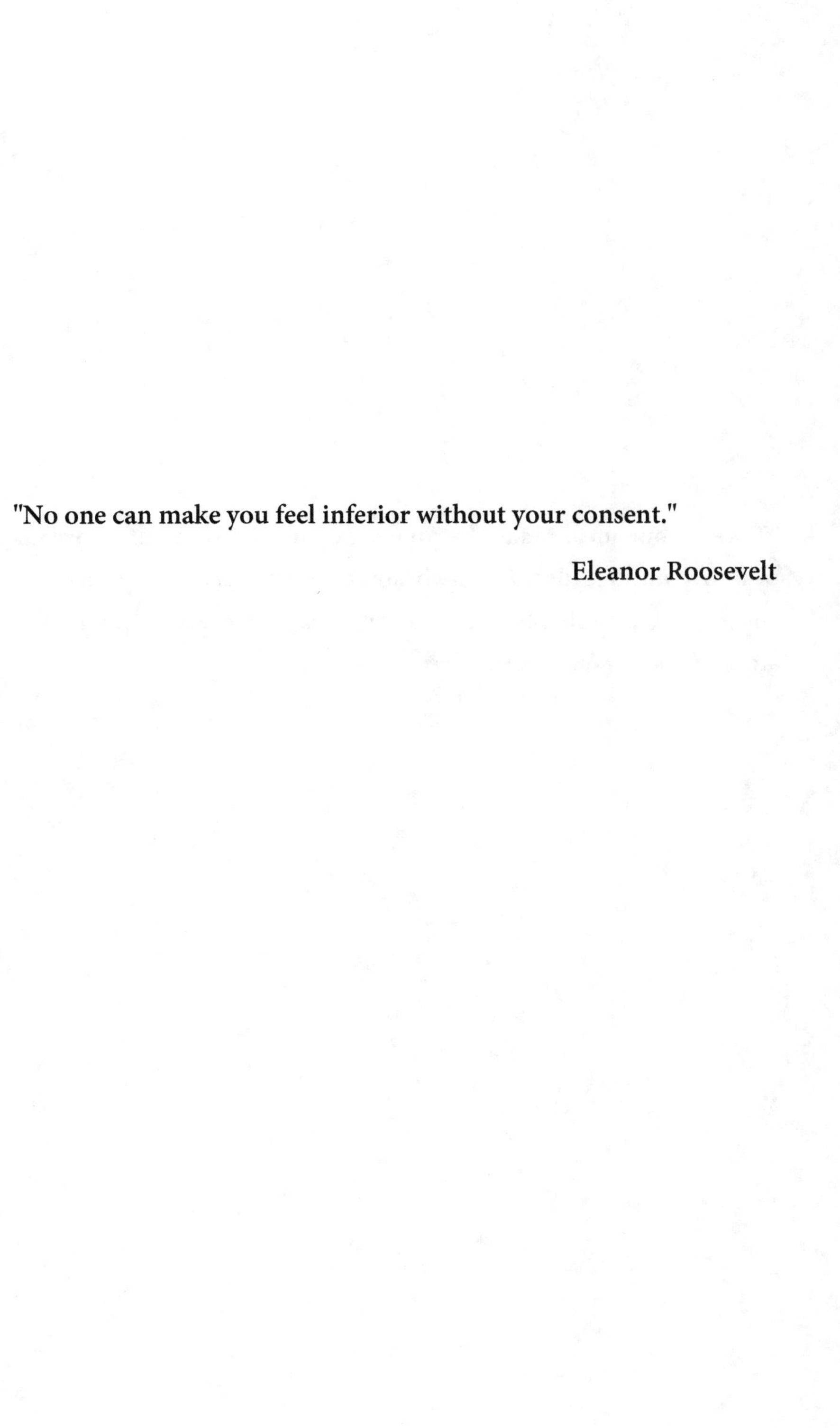

"No one can make you feel inferior without your consent."

Eleanor Roosevelt

"Take up one idea. Make that one idea your life-think of it, dream of it, live on that idea. Let the brain, muscles, nerves, every part of your body, be full of that idea, and just leave every other idea alone. This is the way to success."

Swami Vivekananda

Motivation

Ok so when you hear the word motivation, what comes to your mind? That word actually drains you so let us not use the word motivation. I'm just going to say that I'm going to push you in the right direction. First, find a picture of a person that has your same body frame and height. Second, I want you to find a picture of yourself. Then post these two pictures next to each other on your bathroom mirror. I want you to look at these pictures for at least 2 minutes a day to help remind you that you are going to change. I can't make you change, but you can. I'm giving you the tools so you can push yourself into the right direction. Now drop and give me another 100 pushups. Yes, you heard me loud and clear, and don't get up until you're done and I tell you to recover. Once you're done with the pushups and you recover, we can move to the next part of the business.

Blue Print

It's important to plan your weekly workouts and dieting plan. Without a plan you can't achieve your goals. So write down your plans and don't be lazy and say "Well I can't remember it". That's some straight up bull, so don't do that. One of my favorite quotes is, "You can't manage what you don't measure" So get your gluteus maximus off the couch, get up and let's write our fat melting plan on paper and start your call to action.

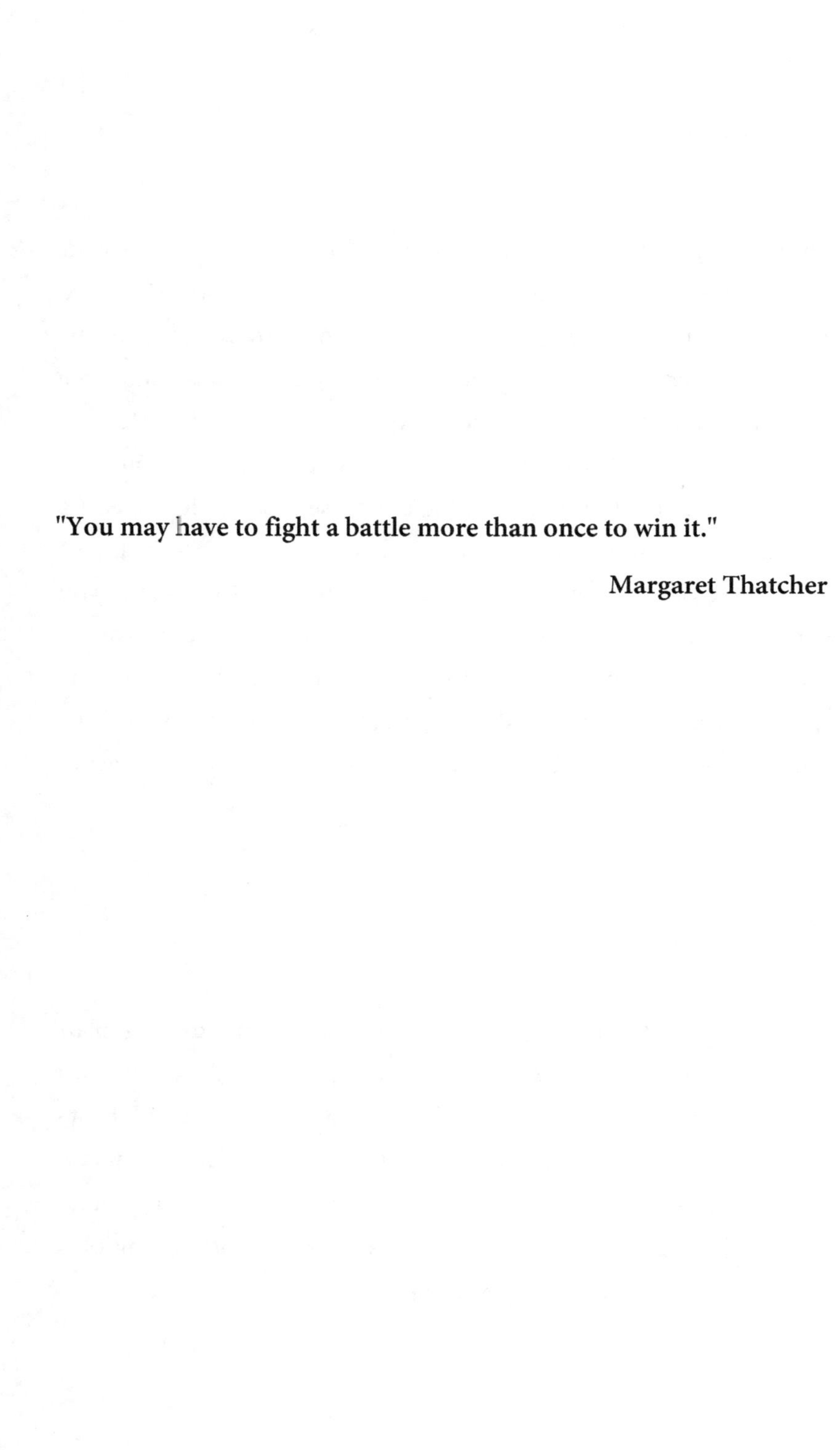

"You may have to fight a battle more than once to win it."

Margaret Thatcher

"Successful and unsuccessful people do not vary greatly in their abilities. They vary in their desires to reach their potential."

John Maxwell

Cleanser

A cleanser helps eliminate toxic waste. Often, our intestines get blocked with materials that have not been eliminated due to of lack of fiber. Yeah EEW! That is a fact. Eating all those hamburgers and pizza contribute to blocked intestines and puts more weight on our bodies. The toxic materials contribute to poor absorption of food, vitamins, and minerals. With the cleanser, you will lose these pounds of toxic waste and you will have a healthier digestive system, a healthier colon, and a lighter body. A good cleanse contributes to nutrient absorption for the body. It is possible, with a healthy diet, that you can lose an extra 1 to 3 pounds.

Natural herbs along with your diet are also beneficial. Natural organic herbs help improve digestion, reduce gas, and relieve intestinal mucus. Natural herbs for cleansing are very powerful. You can use flax seed in your smoothies and shakes. You can also find a good organic whole leaf tea like red raspberry leaf tea to go along with your diet. They help restore and rejuvenate your body. Having a healthy digestive system and colon helps to keep the fat away and maintain a more desirable figure.

Finally, to start your diet plan, read along and remember the following will help give your journey a big boost! So what are you waiting for?

We suggest a body cleanser that eliminates stomach waste and gives you a new fresh start to your new 30-day weight loss program. I recommend warning your friends and family to stay clear for a few days. NOT KIDDING! Here I will give you the recipe and instructions. Make sure to follow the instructions very closely to get the best results. You will lose 10 pounds or more after the seven day cleanse. Remember it is only seven days. Set your mind to it and get it accomplished!

ULTRA-Pro Gut 15-Day Detox

Avoid Sugar and Alcohol for 15 Days. You must eat 5 meals spread out 3-4 hours daily, and drink about gallon of water a day! 1 Cheat Meal a week-is allowed. And no Sugar or Fried foods!

Here is the daily schedule of what to eat plus the supplements;

Meal #1

Unlimited soup

Unlimited Veggies only from the list below (Raw or steamed)

Squash

Tomato

Bell peppers

Green beans

Peas

Cucumber

Asparagus

Carrot

Celery

Lettuce

Drink Unlimited Lemon water

Supplements with Meal#1

Ultra pro-Gut Probiotic 1 pill

Ashwagandha 1 pill

Meal #2

Unlimited soup

Unlimited Veggies only from the list below (Raw or steamed)

Squash

Tomato

Bell peppers

Green beans

Peas

Cucumber

Asparagus

Carrot

Celery

Lettuce

Drink unlimited Lemon Water

Supplements with Meal #2

Ultra pro-Gut Probiotic 1 pill

Ashwagandha 1 pill

Meal #3 Snack

2 scoops Pur-native

Supplements with Meal #3

Ultra pro-Gut Probiotic 1 pill

Ashwagandha 1 pill

Meal #4

Unlimited Soup

Unlimited Veggies only from the list below (Raw or steamed)

Squash

Tomato

Bell peppers

Green beans

Peas

Cucumber

Asparagus

Carrot

Celery

Lettuce

Drink Unlimited Lemon Water

Supplements with Meal #4

Ultra pro-Gut Probiotic 1 pill

Ashwagandha 1 Pill

Meal #5 Snack

Unlimited Cucumbers Add Cayenne pepper and lime juice

Supplements with Meal #5

Ultra pro-Gut Probiotic 1 pill

Ashwagandha 1 pill

Avoid sugar and alcohol!

Drink plenty of water! If you feel dehydrated please add electrolytes to your water this will allow you to be hydrated.

Grocery list of ingredients for Soup

Here is a quick pick up list for the soup;

Organic Chicken Bone broth

Large Onion, Peeled and Chopped

Organic Fresh Broccoli Florets

Chopped Celery

Chopped Parsley

Garlic Cloves, Minced

Fresh shredded or grated ginger

Olive Oil

Crushed red pepper or cayenne pepper

Ground turmeric

Himalayan Pink salt and pepper

Beyond Meat

Shredded chicken

How to make soup

Add the following ingredients in a big Pot.

Slow cook and shred the meat then add to the boiling pot.

*2-4 Quarts Organic Chicken Bone broth

* 1 Large Onion, Peeled and Chopped

* 3 Cups Organic Fresh Broccoli Florets

*3 Cups Chopped Celery

* 1/4 Cup Chopped Parsley

* 4 Garlic Cloves, Minced

* 4 Tablespoon fresh shredded or grated ginger

* 2 tablespoon olive Oil

* 1/4-1/2 teaspoon crushed red pepper or cayenne pepper

* 1/4 teaspoon ground turmeric

* Add Himalayan Pink salt and pepper

Add Beyond Meat (optional if you're vegan)

This will last for 3 days if you ate 5 cups a day!

Add the following ingredients for Organic only

ADD the Shredded chicken

* 1 1/2 Pounds Organic Boneless skinless chicken breast. Shredded chicken (Make in crockpot)

OR

Place chicken breasts into a saucepan and pour in enough water to cover. Place over medium heat, bring to a boil, and simmer until chicken meat is no longer pink, 10 to 12 minutes. Transfer chicken breasts to a bowl, allow to cool, and shred the chicken meat with 2 forks.

For Vegans

ADD Beyond Meat

*1 ½ pounds organic Beyond Meat-Chop up and add in soup

Organic Veggie & Salads

Anything off this list will hurt your weight loss. If it's not on the list, then you can't have it.

Steamed Veggies Only

Squash

Tomato

Bell peppers

Green beans

Peas

Cucumber

Asparagus

Carrot

Celery

Lettuce

Snack

Cucumber –Add Lemon Juice on top and Cayenne Pepper

Dressing- Apple cider Vinegar & Olive Oil – Salt and pepper (Only)

Fresh Herbs

Here is the list of fresh herbs that are useful during your weight loss program.

Basil

Chives

Dill

Oregano

Parsley

Rosemary

Sage

Tarragon

ECT….

Order Supplements online at a discounted rate:

1. Ultra Pro Gut – Help heal stomach - $25.00 Discounted

2. Ashwagandha Adaptogen stress - $15 Discounted

ORDER ONLINE

www.darrickbynum.com

Discount Code - Darrick40

Order Pur native Protein (Not discounted)

https://www.nutristat.com/

"The mark of a great man is one who knows when to set aside the important things in order to accomplish the vital ones."

Brandon Sanderson

"Victory has a hundred fathers and defeat is an orphan."

John F. Kennedy

Diet

Now we have to make a more permanent plan for the rest of your weight loss journey. I'm sure you're like, "Diet? Hahahaha!" Yes, without this it's hard to lose weight, or to transform your body. The key to this is to write down what you eat, count your calories, and make sure that you are eating

5 small meals a day. It's that simple write down what you eat and count your calories. Calories in verses calories out correct? So take your time to write it down and come up with a game plan to eat 5 meals a day. Try to eat veggies and protein for every meal and you will see results. I will include what type of foods you should eat for every meal. Try to only have one dessert a night or, even better, just one on weekends. I tell my clients that working out and dieting is a full-time job, but you have the weekends off and you can enjoy it. You deserve it!

Sometimes you might complain that everything you eat makes you fat. However, it's really your responsibility to learn about healthy foods so that you can eat healthier. Very healthy delicious foods to help you burn fat are fruit smoothies. You can make your own smoothies full of antioxidants with fruits and vegetables. A real healthy smoothie will have about 250 calories in comparison to 500 calories in readymade fast food smoothies. Another source of food you need is protein. For instance, eggs have a lot of protein. Protein helps make you feel full and satisfied for longer. You can eat two eggs with a slice of whole wheat bread.

Fruits and vegetables for salads have low calorie content. Broccoli in salads also helps prevent cancer. Broccoli has calcium, iron, magnesium, vitamin A, and vitamin C. Salads are big in volume, and, therefore, signal your brain to eat less because your eyes see them as a lot of food. You will have higher contents of vitamin C, E, and lycopene if you eat your veggies more often daily. Fruits with a high content of water like melon and cucumbers have lower calories and fill that belly up a lot. Citric fruits have high vitamin C content. These fruits are powerful fat busting fruits. It's a good idea to invest in a really good multivitamin and other daily supplement that you need. Don't be cheap! You also need minerals, and have to invest in a really good source of protein mix. You can try different flavors of protein mixes to add to your shakes or smoothies. A good high-quality protein mix will have low sugar content and will keep that belly of yours satisfied for longer periods.

I recommend that you drink a full 12oz of water before you eat any meal or snack. Drinking enough water helps curb your appetite. Most of the times you think you are hungry when, in reality, you are just dehydrated and the body only wants water. For example, if you have already eaten enough and feel hungry, more often than not, you are actually thirsty. Eating again when you really don't need to is only adding extra calories to your day that are not needed.

Water also keeps your digestive system healthy. Not drinking enough water can also make you feel tired. If your muscles are dehydrated, you will feel tired. Water, along with strength training, helps define and tone your muscles.

You should always consult with your doctor before starting any diet and exercise program. Have your thyroid tested. If you have an undiagnosed hypothyroidism it needs to be treated in order to get best results from your diet program. You need to take a multivitamin, Super B-Complex preferably in liquid, Vitamin C mix, and a daily fiber supplement.

Successful diet foods and routines

No bread for 3 weeks

1-2 cups of coffee or something with high caffeine in the morning

Very little carbs

Sweet potatoes

Protein bars

Oat meal – unflavored

Nuts, almonds

Greek yogurt – 14 grams protein

Steak, chicken breast, lean meat, fish

Cottage cheese

Peanut butter

Fruits, ruby grape fruit, smoothies- add protein

Green vegetables

Liquid Fatty acids

Jell-O (calcium) milk, dairy

Amino acids (GNC) pills

Must get 8 hours of sleep every night; this is crucial to weight loss

Weekly Sample Diet Plan

Monday

Breakfast: Meal Replacement Shake preferably sugar-free, a cup of coffee with no sugar and no milk. Take your multivitamin Vitamin C.

Lunch: Salad. Add nuts, Cube lean turkey chunks in your salad for protein, half a grapefruit. Take your Super B-Complex vitamin

Dinner: Fish, salad, half a grapefruit, plain green tea before bed.

Tuesday

Breakfast: Oatmeal, a cup of coffee with no sugar and no milk. Take your multivitamin Vitamin C.

Lunch: Tuna, salad and half a grapefruit. Take your Super B-Complex vitamin

Dinner: Steak, salad and half a grapefruit, plain green tea before bed.

Wednesday

Breakfast: Cup of coffee with no sugar and no milk. Take your multivitamin Vitamin C.

Lunch: Baked Potato, Half a grapefruit, B Complex Vitamin

Dinner: Salmon, spinach and lettuce salad, and half a grapefruit, plain green tea.

Thursday

Breakfast: Make a healthy smoothie (Skim milk, banana, protein powder mix, berries), a cup of coffee with no sugar and no milk. Take your multivitamin Vitamin C.

Lunch: Brown rice, salad, and half a grapefruit. Take your Super B-Complex vitamin

Dinner: Sirloin, broccoli, and half a grapefruit, plain green tea before bed.

Friday

Breakfast: A cup of coffee with no sugar and no milk. Take your multivitamin Vitamin C.

Lunch: Half a grapefruit. Take your Super B-Complex vitamin
Dinner: Turkey, salad, half a grapefruit, plain green tea before bed.

REMEMBER: Make sure to eat healthy snacks as mentioned to make your 5 small meals a day. Have Greek yogurt, protein bar, and drink as much organic green tea as you want. This will help curb your appetite.

GRAPEFRUITS ARE YOUR FRIENDS!

You are probably wondering why in the sample diet plan I recommend the grapefruit consistently as part of your diet. This is because grapefruits block deposits of fat in your system. They also help the body burn more fat during workouts and help you lose more fat very fast. Grapefruits improve your cardiovascular health. Red and white grapefruits have powerful antioxidants that benefit your heart, and you definitely need a healthy heart to support your workouts. They help oxidize bad nasty cholesterol by

15% and reduce fats that make the heart sick by up to 17 %. You can lose up to three pounds more by eating ½ a grapefruit daily. Eat grapefruit with all your meals. It will boost your metabolism to burn fat faster.

There are certain things you can add to your diet, but only in moderation. For example, there is nothing wrong with using butter, but not frequently. The key to this is moderation, and how often of certain things you should consume. You can use a little butter on vegetables and fry vegetables with butter, but a very little amount. Don't eat pastry and candy. Try all varieties of healthy veggies. Try onions, peppers, carrots and peas, and radishes. Experiment with all the different kinds in your salads or as sides with lean meats.

Now follow me and let's get started with your workout plan. Say in your mind "Working out will make me feel great". Keep that in your mind through the entire day to help you start enjoying working out, because yes, I know sometimes working out is just not one of those things we really like to do, but you might surprise yourself and that might not be the case.

"You have to be burning with an idea, or a problem, or a wrong that you want to right. If you're not passionate enough from the start, you'll never stick it out."

Steve Jobs

"The only way to do great work is to love what you do."

Steve Jobs

Don't Skip Your Workouts!

It's lame to say you are too busy to exercise. The time you spend in front of the tube sitting on the couch, you could exercise.

<u>Workout Plan</u>

Example of 3x10 squats

3 means sets

10 means reps

1 set 10 squats then rest

2nd set 10 squats then rest

3rd set 10 squats then rest

Monday

3x50 jumping jacks morning and night

3x10 squats 20 second rest in sets

Tuesday

3x50 jumping jacks when you wake up

1x50 jumping jacks at lunch time

2x50 jumping jacks at night before bed

Find a workout at home

Wednesday

3x50 jumping jacks

5 x 25 crunches

Thursday

3 x 50 jumping jacks when you wake up

1x50 jumping jacks at lunchtime

2x50 jumping jacks at night before bed

Friday

3 x 50 jumping jacks when you wake up

1x50 Jumping jacks at lunch time

2x50 jumping jacks at night before bed

Saturday

3 x 50 jumping jacks when you wake up

1x50 Jumping jacks at lunch time

4x50 jumping jacks at night before bed

3 x 50 crunches

Sunday - rest

"Much of the stress that people feel doesn't come from having too much to do. It comes from not finishing what they've started."

David Allen

"Focus on the journey, not the destination. Joy is found not in finishing an activity but in doing it."

Greg Anderson

Metabolism & Carbohydrates

Now let's discuss some additional valuable tips to help you on your incredible journey towards a thinner new you. It's possible to increase your metabolism. It will help you to tone your muscles, and in building more muscle. Muscle cells are more active than fat cells and burn more calories than fat. It's very important that you drink enough water to maintain your muscles by keeping them properly hydrated. Drinking enough water helps your body maintain the right body temperature, which in turn prevents extra storing of fat. Physical activity helps boosts metabolism for several hours after a workout. Therefore, during your resting metabolic rate your muscles continue to burn more calories to repair and recover.

Carbohydrates are important in the building of muscle. Eating carbs help replenish your glycogen. You use glycogen as energy during your workout. Carbohydrates come in simple sugars such as glucose and sucrose, and complex carbohydrates.

When you eat these simple carbs/sugars they get digested and absorbed into your body very quickly. The problem with this is you will start craving more sugar. Which we all know will make you gain weight quickly. Try keeping your simple carbs intake in the form of only fruit, vegetables, and dairy.

Complex carbs such as whole grains breads, potatoes, and beans, on the other hand, take much longer to break down into sugar in your body. The unprocessed grains in complex carbs contain fiber that will keep you fuller for longer periods and help you move waste out of your body.

There are many good sugar substitutes out there. You just have to find the one that is right for you. There are also little sugar free treats that you can buy that are very tasty without the sugar blues attached. Finding a decent sugar substitute is one of the simplest ways to lose weight because you really don't have to change too much.

WARNING: STAY AWAY FROM THE FOLLOWING SIMPLE CARBS!

Chocolate

Soft Drinks

Cakes

Biscuits

White bread / White rice

"You get in life what you have the courage to ask for."

Nancy D. Solomon

"Wisdom equals knowledge plus courage. You have to not only know what to do and when to do it, but you have to also be brave enough to follow through."

Jarod Kintz

Strength Training

Strength training protects your bone health and muscle mass. As you get older you begin to lose about 1% of your bone and muscle strength ever year. Adding strength training to your workout helps prevent this.

Strength training makes you stronger and fitter. Strength training is also called resistance training because it involves strengthening and toning your muscles by contracting them against a resisting force. Resistance exercise can raise metabolic rate, an important factor in maintaining body weight.

Remember that with strength training your muscles need time to recover, so you should only do it to certain body parts on alternate days. Make sure you always warm up before and cool down after strength training.

Strength training helps you develop better body mechanics. Strength training has benefits that go well beyond the appearance of nicely toned muscles. Your balance and coordination will improve, as will your posture. More importantly, if you have poor flexibility and balance, strength training can reduce your risk of falling by as much as 40 percent, a crucial benefit, especially as you get older.

It's important that you use the right dumbbells for your strength training workouts. You have to challenge your muscles. If you do 10 repetitions and they seem easy then the weight you're using is too light, but if you struggle on your tenth repetition you are using the correct weight amount. Good for you!

The benefits of weight training include greater muscular strength, improved muscle tone and appearance, increased endurance, and enhanced bone density. It also helps stimulate the cardiovascular system. It helps raise levels of dopamine, serotonin, and norepinephrine, which can help improve mood and counter feelings of depression. How's that for a natural high?

There are two types of weight lifting

Isometric resistance: involves contracting your muscles against a non- moving object, such as against the floor in a push-up.

Isotonic strength training: involves contracting your muscles through a range of motion as in weight lifting.

Foods to include with your Strength Training

Protein Sources:

Fish

Tuna (salmon, perch, haddock)

Turkey

Chicken

Lean Red Meats

Soybeans, legumes, nuts

Carbohydrates: Brown Rice Whole Grains

Vegetables (carrots, broccoli, green beans, corn)

Fat Sources: Olive oil Peanuts Almonds Avocadoes

"In the end, it is important to remember that we cannot become what we need to be by remaining what we are."

Max De Pree

"Whenever you see a successful person, you only see the public glories, never the private sacrifices to reach them."

Vaibhav Shah

MORE VEGGIES, LESS GREASY FOOD

You now have many tools I told you I would help you with. Remember you have a full list of healthy foods you can mix and experiment with. Eating doesn't have to be made boring by eating the same things all the time. You can modify these sample diets with more of the foods that are listed. Try nuts on your salads, mix different vegetables with meats, and try experimenting with different vegetable and fruit juices. This was more to help push you in a healthier route and get you to your goals. Remember to write everything down in your diet journal. Even if you miss your workouts write it in your journal to help remind you to do better. It is hard to stay on track with dieting and working out at the beginning, but the more you work out, the more you are going to WANT to work out.

Another thing is eating healthy. The more good powerful healthy foods you eat, the more you are going to want to eat healthier foods. You are probably thinking how that can be? It's true that grease makes certain foods taste better but when your body sticks to high-quality healthy foods it will start desiring to eat that way. Your body will want less of the foods that give you that muffin top and double chin.

Here are some tips to help in your weight loss journey

Clean your closet of the "fat" clothes. Once you've reached your target weight, throw out or give away every piece of clothing that doesn't fit. The idea of having to buy a completely new wardrobe if you gain the weight back will serve as a strong incentive to maintain your new figure.

Once a week, indulge in a high-calorie-tasting, but low-calorie, treat. This should help keep you from feeling deprived and binging on higher-calorie foods.

Buy a pedometer, clip it to your belt, and aim for an extra 1,000 steps a day. Skip the ride and take a walk. Walking only 15 minutes each day burns more than 40 calories. A casual daily walk could burn more than four pounds in a year. Use the mall stairs while shopping instead of elevators or escalators to reduce weight even more. The calories from snacks quickly add up to extra pounds. Keep a snack diary and record the times when you snack the most. Find a new hobby during those times or make sure you have a healthy snack at hand.

Purchase low-calorie substitute snacks to replace high-calorie alternatives. Popcorn, celery, and carrot sticks are low-calorie alternatives to high- calorie snacks such as potato chips and cookies.

Developing an outdoor hobby is a way to integrate exercise with a high- interest activity. An hour of gardening burns more than

300 calories. Fast-food meals and snacks come loaded with calories, not to mention unhealthy fats and chemicals. Having a naughty meal once or twice a week is fine and should be seen as a reward for your hard work. Never cut your favorite foods out of your diet or you'll cave in eventually and eat them by the bucket. Plan to have your favorites once or twice a week to have something to look forward to. This solution really works, because you never really go without.

Bring only enough money to purchase only one select food item; this keeps calorie intake to a minimum. Let friends know that fast food is off the diet and make a list of alternative, healthy dining locations for afterschool or weekend outings.

Don't find the closest park; instead find one that makes you walk a little further. Don't be lazy! C'mon! Use those legs!

Get out in the fresh air often. It invigorates the body and mind with its purity, and can energize you to walk or run. Don't stay inside cooped up like a farmhouse chicken, get out alive, burn fat, and lose weight. Have fun!

There are many good sugar substitutes out there. You just have to find the one that is right for you. There are also little sugar free treats that you can buy, that are very tasty without the sugar blues attached. Finding a decent sugar substitute is one of the simplest ways to lose weight because you really don't have to change too much.

YOU CAN GET THE RESULTS YOU WANT

After thirty days, I want you to look back at the picture that we talked about at the beginning of the program, and I want you to stare at it, and see the amazing results you have achieved. I have faith in the fact that you got tough, stuck it out, and just did it. Sometimes you just have to do something you might not want to at first in order to realize you want to do it and will learn to like it. In this case, you will learn to like working out, and yes, eating healthy.

Keep you gluteus maximus off the couch and stay away from evil muffins and in return you will see a sexier new you!

"It is not the strongest of the species that survive, nor the most intelligent, but the one most responsive to change."

Charles Darwin

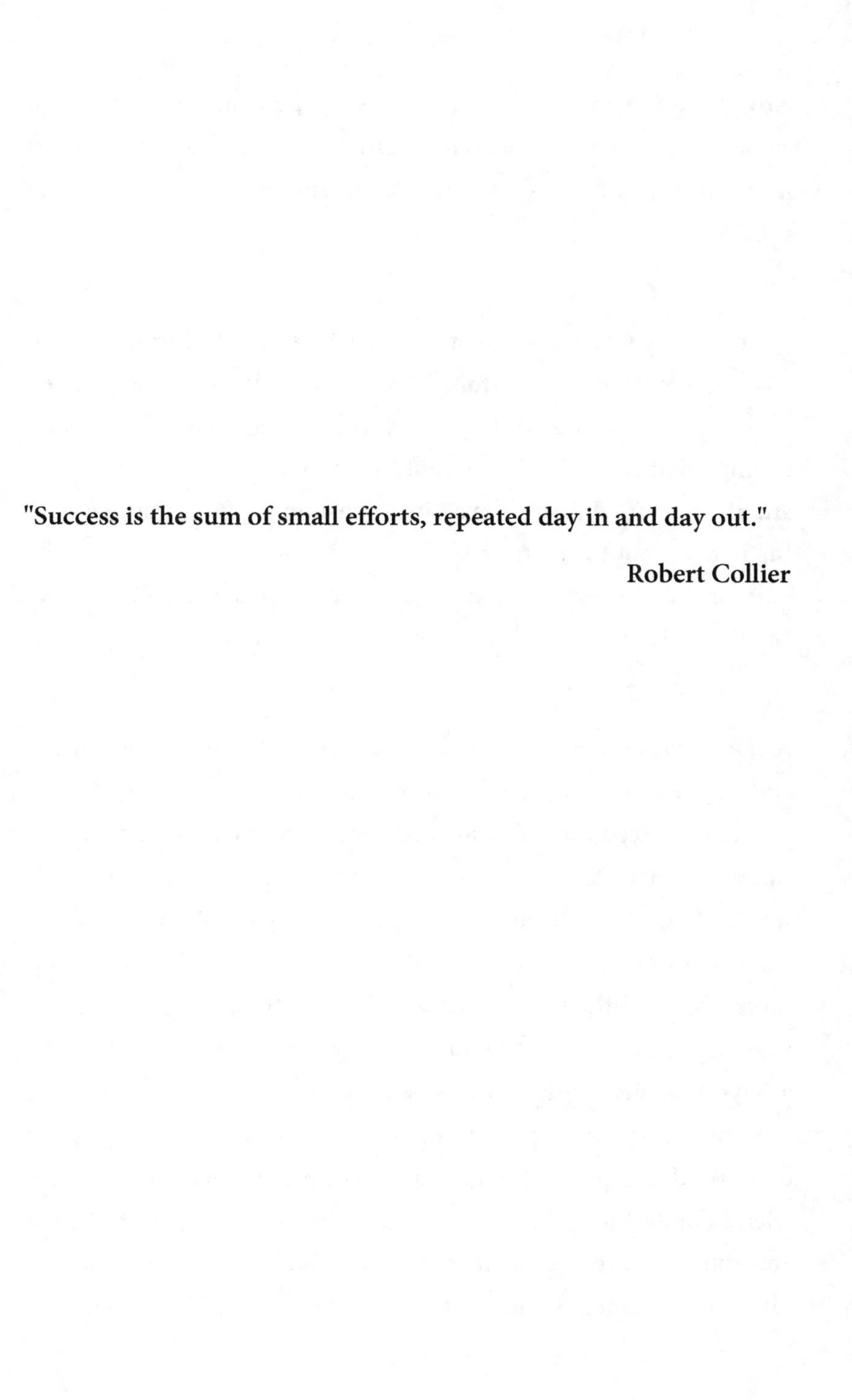

"Success is the sum of small efforts, repeated day in and day out."

Robert Collier

Now I want you to read the following personal account from someone that achieved amazing results. His goals and success can help push you to take action, to pursue your own goals and succeed!

"Within only 90 days, I, Jonathan Kuthe went from 280 pounds to 234 pounds. That is an astonishing 46 pounds lost. What helped me get through the 90 days was setting a big goal. I did this by having smaller goals throughout the month that I knew I can attain, adding different exercises, pushing myself harder and further. Without a plan you have nothing. I saw myself losing 30 pounds, but I over achieved that. Darrick taught me how to make small weekly goals and I surpassed every one of them.

As far as my diet goes I try to limit portion sizes, trying new fruits and veggies, cooking my foods by eliminating seasoning, butter, and oils. I forced myself to workout. I can't even tell you how many times I wanted to not workout, but I saw my weekly goal, and I wanted to beat that. That's what kept me going. I realized that when I had nothing to do, all I wanted to do was eat. So I had to keep myself busy all the time. Whenever I had nothing to do I used that time as an opportunity to go to the gym and work out. Darrick always kept me motivated. I was truly blessed to have him there every step of the way. I can tell you this much, it is worth every penny to have the support I received. I recommend having a coach, friends, and fitness club that has the same goals as you do. It was amazing to have people that actually care about you, and not push you for money. I'm telling you, I don't care what state or city you live in you need to come to the Darrick Bynum Health & Wellness Center in Wood Dale. I couldn't have lost the 46 pounds on my own without the support of them. Having a group of people working out with me with the same transformation goals was great not having to worry about who is watching you or laughing at you. Making new friends made it fun that much more to workout. I'm not trying to sell you Darrick Bynum Health & Wellness Center, not at all because that's not what they are about. Darrick Bynum Health & Wellness Center stands for fighting your way fit. P90X and The Biggest Loser have nothing on Darrick Bynum. He has the skills to motivate you and get you to where you want to be. There are many great trainers out there, but very few that can motivate you to want this, and have fun while you're doing it. I never thought I would love working out but Darrick Bynum Health & Wellness Center changed all that. I love to work out now. I run 5-10 miles a day! Wow! It's crazy even saying that because I used to struggle running only a block.

I just signed up for the Chicago Men's Health Urbanathlon. This is my lifestyle now, because I want a healthier life style. My friend, you have to take this as a lifestyle change and don't think of it as a diet, or you will fail. Every day is a challenge and that's why I signed up at the Darrick Bynum Health & Wellness Center. They keep me motivated and keep me on my feet. Trust me when you first start the program it's going to be hard. Yes, your family loves you and supports you, but they are going to eat and drink whatever they want in front of you. Don't get caught up in that, stay focused and connect with positive people that have the same goals as you. Don't get discouraged when you drive to work and see

McDonalds, Dairy Queen, or the billboards with food and beer on them. Trust me; I still struggle with that addiction of beer and food. I admit it, I have a problem, but I can overcome that, it's my fight not my family's. Keep in mind you're not going to be a model right away. You didn't put the weight on overnight; it was a process. Try to avoid having cheat days or slipping up. I know in the back of your mind you say, "Well, I can work it off " Stop! That has failure written all over it. Just don't do it!

Stay focused on the prize. Stay far away from people who drink. I'm telling you, I slipped and it cost me a setback. Don't do it, your will power is not that strong. If you have to go to an event, eat before you go. Also weigh yourself first. This helped me a lot for my birthday and some other events that I went to.

I love working out now! There are times I just don't want to, but I make myself, and after I do I feel great! So I wish you all the best on your transformation!

I want to say thank you to Sue Turco, Vicky La Voie, Darrick Bynum, Afrim Ramani and the Darrick Bynum Health & Wellness Family. Without all of you, I wouldn't have been able to accomplish what I have!"

Testimonials

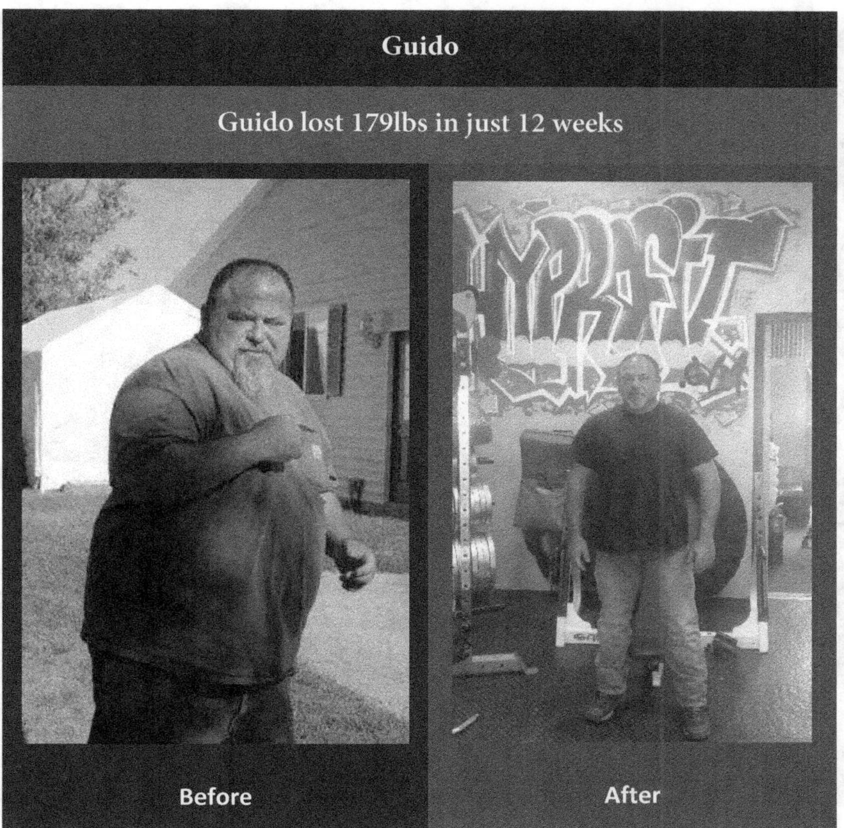

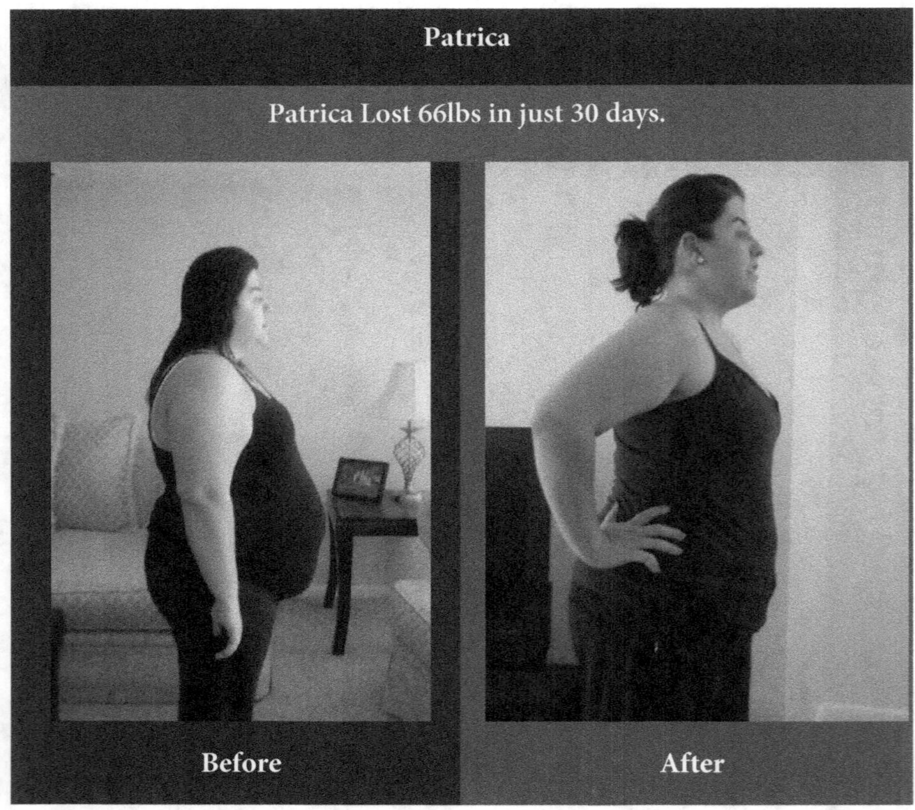

Patrica
Patrica Lost 66lbs in just 30 days.
Before
After

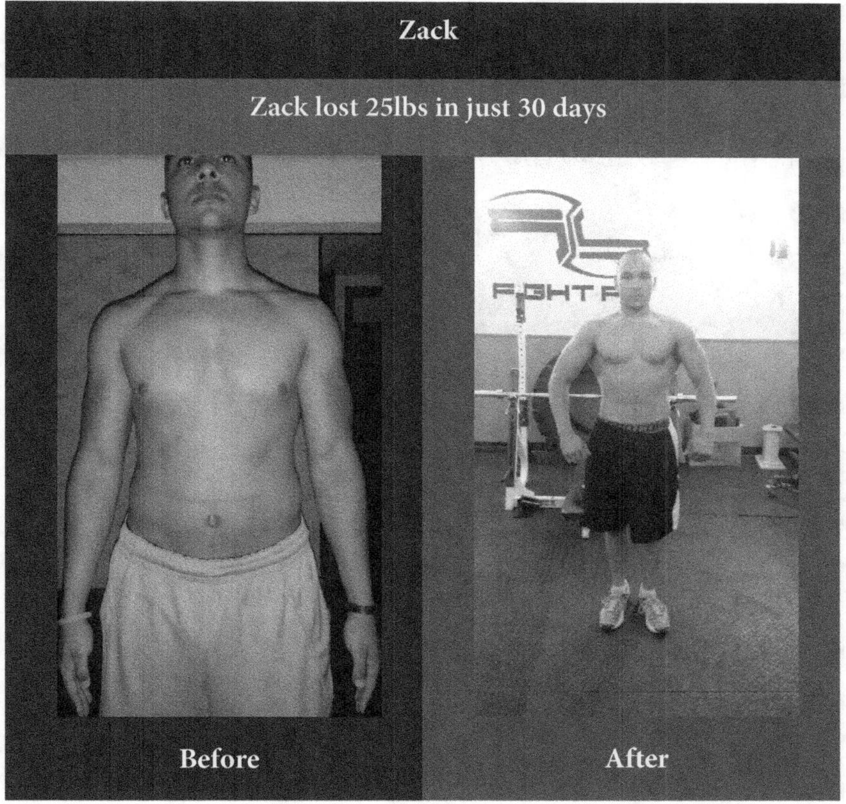
Zack
Zack lost 25lbs in just 30 days
Before
After

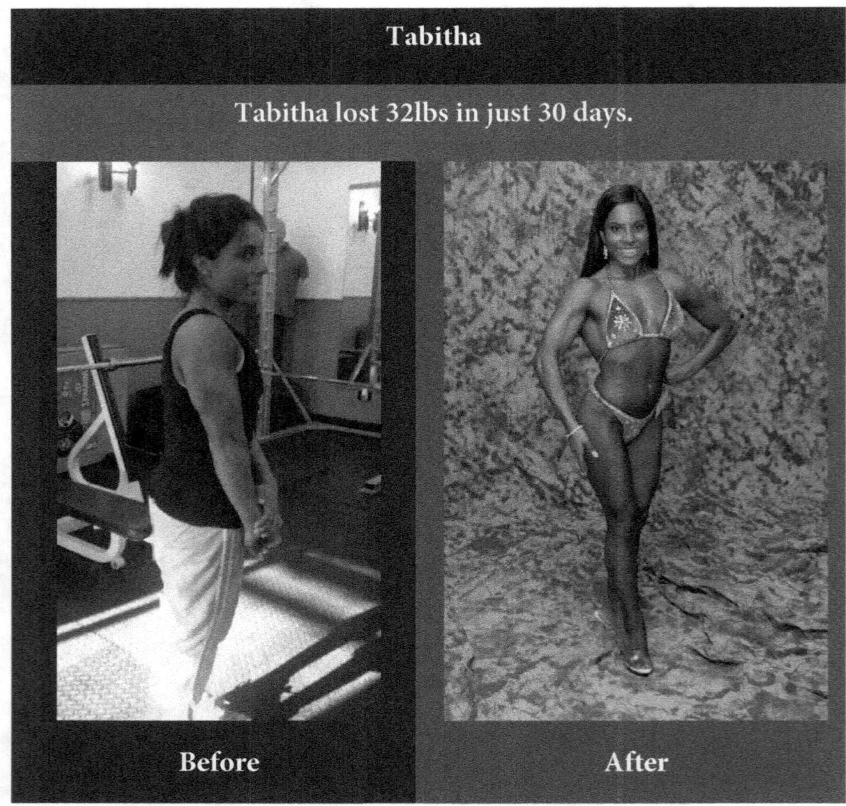

Tabitha
Tabitha lost 32lbs in just 30 days.
Before
After

"If you are willing to do more than you are paid to do,
eventually you will be paid to do more than you do."

Anonymous

Beginners

30 Day

Home Workout Program

"Success is walking from failure to failure with no loss of enthusiasm."

Winston Churchill

Day 1

Monday

Exercise	Reps	Sets	Rest
Jumping Jacks	5	3	30 seconds
Squats	5	3	30 seconds
Alternating Lunges	5 per side	3	30 seconds
Crunches	5	3	30 seconds

"Try not to become a person of success, but rather try to become a person of value."

Albert Einstein

Day 2

Tuesday

Exercise	Reps	Sets	Rest
Jumping Jacks	6	3	30 seconds
Squats	6	3	30 seconds
Alternating Lunges	5 per side	3	30 seconds
Crunches	6	3	30 seconds

"Great minds discuss ideas; average minds discuss events; small minds discuss people."

Eleanor Roosevelt

Day 3

Wednesday

Exercise	Reps	Sets	Rest
Jumping Jacks	7	3	30 seconds
Squats	7	3	30 seconds
Alternating Lunges	5 per side	3	30 seconds
Crunches	7	3	30 seconds

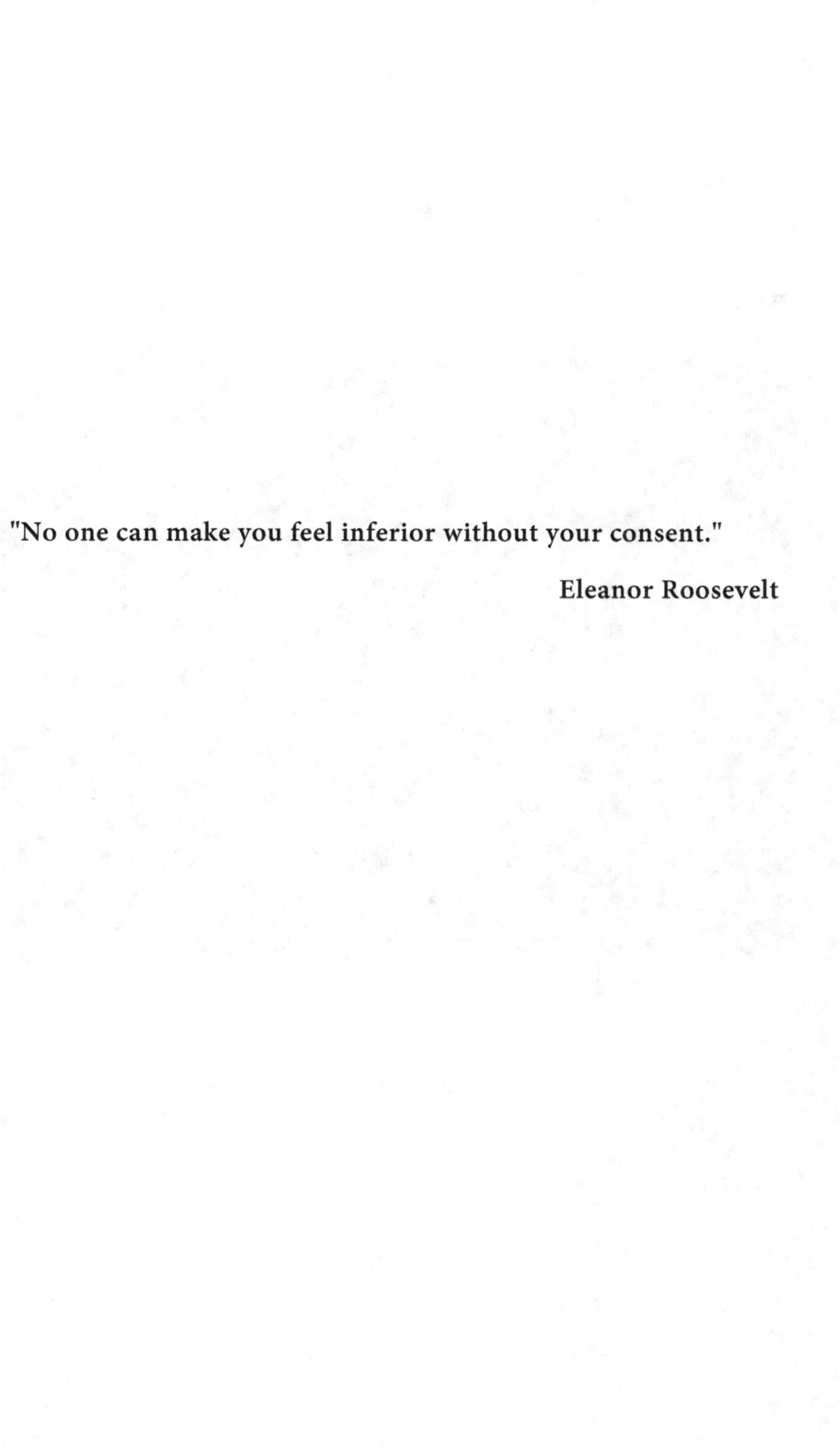

"No one can make you feel inferior without your consent."

Eleanor Roosevelt

Day 4

Thursday

Exercise	Reps	Sets	Rest
Jumping Jacks	8	3	30 seconds
Squats	8	3	30 seconds
Alternating Lunges	5 per side	3	30 seconds
Crunches	10	3	30 seconds

"The distance between insanity and genius is measured only by success."

Bruce Feirstein

Day 5

Friday

Exercise	Reps	Sets	Rest
Jumping Jacks	10	3	30 seconds
Squats	10	3	30 seconds
Alternating Lunges	5 per side	3	30 seconds
Crunches	15	3	30 seconds

"Don't be afraid to give up the good to go for the great."

John D. Rockefeller

Day 6

Saturday

Exercise	Reps	Sets	Rest
Jumping Jacks	11	3	30 seconds
Squats	12	3	30 seconds
Alternating Lunges	5 per side	3	30 seconds
Crunches	18	3	30 seconds

"There are two types of people who will tell you that you cannot make a difference in this world: those who are afraid to try and those who are afraid you will succeed."

Ray Goforth

Day 7

Sunday

Exercise	Reps	Sets	Rest
REST			
REST			
REST			
REST			

REST

"Courage is resistance to fear, mastery of fear -- not absence of fear."

Mark Twain

Day 8

Monday

Exercise	Reps	Sets	Rest
Jumping Jacks	20	4	30 seconds
Squats	13	3	30 seconds
Alternating Lunges	6 per side	3	30 seconds
Crunches	20	3	30 seconds
Jog in Place	20 sec	3	30 seconds

"Only put off until tomorrow what you are willing to die having left undone."

Pablo Picasso

Day 9

Tuesday

Exercise	Reps	Sets	Rest
Jumping Jacks	21	4	30 seconds
Squats	14	3	30 seconds
Alternating Lunges	6 per side	3	30 seconds
Crunches	25	3	30 seconds
Jog in Place	20 sec	3	30 seconds

"Twenty years from now, you will be more disappointed by the things that you didn't do than by the ones you did do. So throw off the bowlines. Sail away from the safe harbor. Catch the trade winds in your sails. Explore. Dream. Discover."

Mark Twain

Day 10

Wednesday

Exercise	Reps	Sets	Rest
Jumping Jacks	24	4	30 seconds
Squats	15	3	30 seconds
Alternating Lunges	6 per side	3	30 seconds
Crunches	30	3	30 seconds
Jog in Place	20 sec	3	30 seconds

"The successful warrior is the average man, with laserlike focus."

Bruce Lee

Day 11

Thursday

Exercise	Reps	Sets	Rest
Jumping Jacks	25	4	30 seconds
Squats	16	3	30 seconds
Alternating Lunges	6 per side	3	30 seconds
Crunches	30	3	30 seconds
Jog in Place	20 sec	3	30 seconds

"You can't connect the dots looking forward; you can only connect them looking backward. So you have to trust that the dots will somehow connect in your future. You have to trust in something -- your gut, destiny, life, karma, whatever. This approach has never let me down, and it has made all the difference in my life."

Steve Jobs

Day 12

Friday

Exercise	Reps	Sets	Rest
Jumping Jacks	28	4	30 seconds
Squats	17	3	30 seconds
Alternating Lunges	6 per side	3	30 seconds
Crunches	30	3	30 seconds
Jog in Place	20 sec	3	30 seconds

"Successful people do what unsuccessful people are not willing to do. Don't wish it were easier; wish you were better."

Jim Rohn

Day 13

Saturday

Exercise	Reps	Sets	Rest
Jumping Jacks	30	4	30 seconds
Squats	17	3	30 seconds
Alternating Lunges	6 per side	3	30 seconds
Crunches	30	3	30 seconds
Jog in Place	20 sec	3	30 seconds

"The No. 1 reason people fail in life is because they listen to their friends, family, and neighbors."

Napoleon Hill

Day 14

Sunday

Exercise	Reps	Sets	Rest
REST			
REST			
REST			
REST			
REST			

REST

"Many of life's failures are people who did not realize how close they were to success when they gave up."

Thomas A. Edison

Day 15

Monday

Exercise	Reps	Sets	Rest
Jumping Jacks	35	4	30 seconds
Squats	18	3	30 seconds
Alternating Lunges	7 per side	3	30 seconds
Crunches	40	3	30 seconds
Jog in Place	20 sec	3	30 seconds
Planks	10 sec	3	30 seconds

"What would you attempt to do if you knew you would not fail?"

Robert Schuller

Day 16

Tuesday

Exercise	Reps	Sets	Rest
Jumping Jacks	36	4	30 seconds
Squats	19	3	30 seconds
Alternating Lunges	8 per side	3	30 seconds
Crunches	45	3	30 seconds
Jog in Place	25 sec	3	30 seconds
Planks	10 sec	3	30 seconds

"Always bear in mind that your own resolution to success is more important than any other one thing."

Abraham Lincoln

Day 17

Wednesday

Exercise	Reps	Sets	Rest
Jumping Jacks	37	4	30 seconds
Squats	20	3	30 seconds
Alternating Lunges	9 per side	3	30 seconds
Crunches	50	3	30 seconds
Jog in Place	25 sec	3	30 seconds
Planks	10 sec	3	30 seconds

"Do what you have always done and you'll get what you have always got."

Sue Knight

Day 18

Thursday

Exercise	Reps	Sets	Rest
Jumping Jacks	40	4	30 seconds
Squats	20	3	30 seconds
Alternating Lunges	9 per side	3	30 seconds
Crunches	50	3	30 seconds
Jog in Place	25 sec	3	30 seconds
Planks	10 sec	3	30 seconds

"Keep your fears to yourself, but share your courage with
others."

Robert Louis Stevenson

Day 19

Friday

Exercise	Reps	Sets	Rest
Jumping Jacks	40	4	30 seconds
Squats	22	3	30 seconds
Alternating Lunges	9 per side	3	30 seconds
Crunches	55	3	30 seconds
Jog in Place	25 sec	3	30 seconds
Planks	10 sec	3	30 seconds

"I cannot trust a man to control others who cannot control himself."

Robert E. Lee

Day 20

Saturday

Exercise	Reps	Sets	Rest
Jumping Jacks	45	4	30 seconds
Squats	25	3	30 seconds
Alternating Lunges	9 per side	3	30 seconds
Crunches	55	3	30 seconds
Jog in Place	25 sec	3	30 seconds
Planks	10 sec	3	30 seconds

"In a battle between two ideas, the best one doesn't necessarily win. No, the idea that wins is the one with the most fearless heretic behind it."

Seth Godin

Day 21

Sunday

Exercise	Reps	Sets	Rest
Plank	30 seconds	4	30 seconds
Squats	30	3	30 seconds
Reverse Lunge	5 per side	3	30 seconds
Toe Crunches	3	3	30 seconds
Sprint in place	10 sec	3	30 seconds
Side planks	10 sec	3	30 seconds
Jump Squats	3	3	30 seconds

"Leadership is an action, not a position."

Donald McGannon

Day 22

Monday

Exercise	Reps	Sets	Rest
Plank	30 seconds	4	30 seconds
Squats	35	3	30 seconds
Reverse Lunge	5 per side	3	30 seconds
Toe Crunches	4	3	30 seconds
Sprint in place	15 sec	3	30 seconds
Side planks	10 sec	3	30 seconds
Jump Squats	4	3	30 seconds

"A man always has two reasons for doing anything: a good reason and the real reason."

J.P. Morgan

Day 23

Tuesday

Exercise	Reps	Sets	Rest
Plank	30 seconds	4	30 seconds
Squats	38	3	30 seconds
Reverse Lunge	6 per side	3	30 seconds
Toe Crunches	4	3	30 seconds
Sprint in place	15 sec	3	30 seconds
Side planks	10 sec	3	30 seconds
Jump Squats	4	3	30 seconds

"Whenever you see a successful business, someone once made a courageous decision."

Peter F. Drucker

Day 24

Wednesday

Exercise	Reps	Sets	Rest
Plank	30 seconds	4	30 seconds
Squats	40	3	30 seconds
Reverse Lunge	7 per side	3	30 seconds
Toe Crunches	4	3	30 seconds
Sprint in place	15 sec	3	30 seconds
Side planks	10 sec	3	30 seconds
Jump Squats	4	3	30 seconds
Jumping Jacks	50	3	30 seconds

"A good plan violently executed now is better than a perfect plan executed next week."

George Patton

Day 25

Thursday

Exercise	Reps	Sets	Rest
Plank	30 seconds	4	30 seconds
Squats	41	3	30 seconds
Reverse Lunge	8 per side	3	30 seconds
Toe Crunches	10	3	30 seconds
Sprint in place	20 sec	3	30 seconds
Side planks	15 sec	3	30 seconds
Jump Squats	5	3	30 seconds
Jumping Jacks	60	3	30 seconds

"Low self-confidence isn't a life sentence. Self-confidence can be learned, practiced, and mastered-just like any other skill. Once you master it, everything in your life will change for the better."

Barrie Davenport

Day 26

Friday

Exercise	Reps	Sets	Rest
Plank	30 seconds	4	30 seconds
Squats	42	3	30 seconds
Reverse Lunge	8 per side	3	30 seconds
Toe Crunches	15	4	30 seconds
Sprint in place	20 sec	3	30 seconds
Side planks	15 sec	3	30 seconds
Jump Squats	8	3	30 seconds
Jumping Jacks	70	3	30 seconds

"Do it or not. There is no try."

Yoda

Day 27

Saturday

Exercise	Reps	Sets	Rest
Plank	30 seconds	4	30 seconds
Squats	45	3	30 seconds
Reverse Lunge	8 per side	3	30 seconds
Toe Crunches	17	4	30 seconds
Sprint in place	20 sec	3	30 seconds
Side planks	15 sec	3	30 seconds
Jump Squats	8	3	30 seconds
Jumping Jacks	75	3	30 seconds

"The question isn't who is going to let me; it's who is going to stop me."

Ayn Rand

Day 28

Sunday

Exercise	Reps	Sets	Rest
Plank	30 seconds	4	30 seconds
Squats	50	3	30 seconds
Reverse Lunge	8 per side	3	30 seconds
Toe Crunches	18	4	30 seconds
Sprint in place	20 sec	3	30 seconds
Side planks	15 sec	3	30 seconds
Jump Squats	9	3	30 seconds
Jumping Jacks	80	3	30 seconds

"You wouldn't worry so much about what others think of you
if you realized how seldom they do."

Eleanor Roosevelt

Day 29

Monday

Exercise	Reps	Sets	Rest
Plank	30 seconds	4	30 seconds
Squats	50	3	30 seconds
Reverse Lunge	8 per side	3	30 seconds
Toe Crunches	19	4	30 seconds
Sprint in place	20 sec	3	30 seconds
Side planks	15 sec	3	30 seconds
Jump Squats	10	3	30 seconds
Jumping Jacks	85	3	30 seconds

"The best revenge is massive success."

Frank Sinatra

Day 30

Tuesday

Exercise	Reps	Sets	Rest
Plank	40 seconds	4	30 seconds
Squats	55	3	30 seconds
Reverse Lunge	10 per side	3	30 seconds
Toe Crunches	30	4	30 seconds
Sprint in place	30 sec	3	30 seconds
Side planks	20 sec	3	30 seconds
Jump Squats	10	3	30 seconds
Jumping Jacks	10	3	30 seconds

Congratulations

Contact us

Email: Hyprofitstaff@gmail.com

TRANSFORMATION CENTER

Darrick Bynum Health & Wellness Center

325 W Irving Park Rd Wood dale IL 60191

Website

www.Darrickbynum.com

Order Supplements

Ultra Pro Gut Probiotic - $25.00 Discounted   Code Darrick40
Ashwagandha- $15.00 Discounted Code Darrick40

www.ingramcontent.com/pod-product-compliance
Lightning Source LLC
Chambersburg PA
CBHW050922260726
48660CB00001B/343